FERTILITY CHALLENGE: A SIMPLE REMEDY

SHARON ROBER

Table of Contents

Introduction

Laura and David once lived in a busy metropolis where dreams appeared to flourish. They were profoundly in love, their link strengthened by shared laughter, future ambitions, and an unsaid pledge to start a family together.

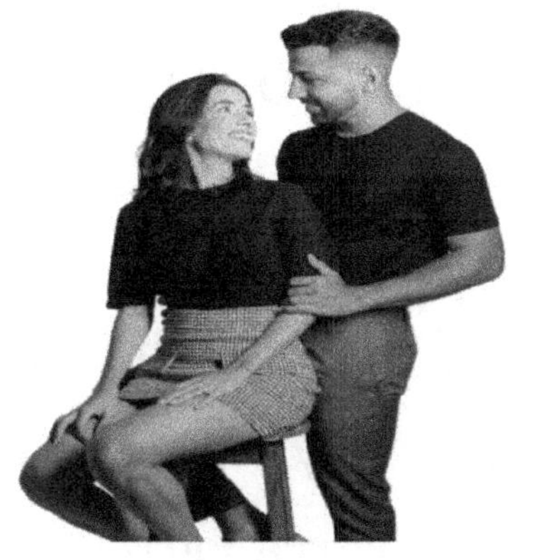

But as the months turned into years, their once bright-eyed optimism faded in the shadow of a hidden struggle: the enormous obstacle of infertility.

Their trip began with enthusiastic expectations, filled with romantic ideas of baby showers and nursery decorations. However, as time passed like sand through an hourglass, their hopes began to fade. Month after month, the joy of potential became the anguish of failure, with each negative pregnancy test a silent echo of unrealized dreams.

Laura and David set out on a mission with heavy hearts and tear-stained cheeks, not for riches or glory, but for the elusive answer to a question that plagued their every thought: why? Why were they unable to conceive? What unseen force stood between them and the family they so dearly wanted?

Their trek took them down meandering routes, through a maze of medical offices and conflicting counsel.

They probed the depths of their bodies, seeking solace in the arms of experts who offered answers but frequently left them with more questions than before.

Despite the uncertainty and sorrow, a glimmer of hope lingered - a notion that somewhere, somehow, there existed a simple solution, a key to unlock the door to their dreams.

This belief drove their determination, initiating a fire within their spirits as they explored deeper into the worlds of science and holistic therapy.

They devoured all knowledge, from the complex workings of the human body to ancient wisdom passed down through centuries.

Their resolve grew stronger with each discovery, and their faith stood firm in the face of adversity.

And then, one fateful day, as the sun bathed the sky in gold and amber, they came across a revelation - a simple solution concealed in plain sight, patiently waiting to be discovered.

It wasn't a miracle cure or a magical potion, but rather a combination of education, lifestyle modifications, and a deeper awareness of themselves.

Laura and David set off on a new chapter of their adventure, full of hope and drive, armed with their acquired understanding. They accepted the challenge before them, knowing that with each step forward, they were one step closer to achieving their goals.

Dear reader, whether you are at the start of your fertility journey or midway along the way, remember that you are not alone.

This book contains a wealth of knowledge, wisdom, and inspiration, as well as a road map to help you navigate the obstacles and victories that await you. So take comfort, since your tale is yet to be told, and everything is conceivable inside its pages.

Chapter 1:

The Science Behind Fertility: Exploring Causes and Factors

Once at a time, in the intricate tapestry of human existence, there was a fundamental urge deep within us to create life, nurture it, and watch it develop.

However, for many, this trip is riddled with difficulties and barriers that stand between them and the fulfillment of their truest desire.

In this chapter, we'll look at the deep science of fertility, peeling back the layers of complexity to reveal the hidden realities that form our knowledge of conception.

From the delicate dance of hormones to the enigmatic workings of the reproductive system, we go on a voyage of discovery, driven by the light of knowledge and fueled by curiosity.

At the core of fertility is a symphony of hormones, each of which plays an important part in orchestrati ng the complex process of conception

.

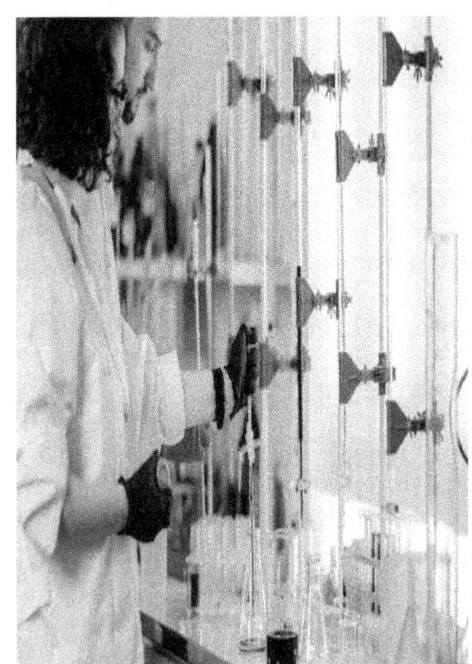

From the throbbing rhythm of the menstrual cycle to the surge of ovulation, hormonal

cues serve as the foundation for the miracle of life.

However, like a delicate equilibrium, the slightest disruption can send ripples across this perfect song, posing obstacles in conception.

However, hormones are only one element of the issue. To uncover the secrets of fertility, we must investigate the numerous elements that influence our reproductive health. Lifestyle decisions, environmental exposures, genetics, and age all have a significant impact on our fertility journey.

As we delve deeper into the maze of reproductive science, we come across harsh realities that many people confront, such as polycystic ovarian syndrome (PCOS), endometriosis, and male factor infertility, each with its own set of problems to conquer.

However, armed with information and wisdom, we may cross these perilous waters with grace and fortitude.

Again, amidst the hardships, there are moments of triumph, stories of perseverance, and optimism that motivate us to persevere in the face of adversity.

From the couple who overcame the chances to conceive against all odds to innovative research that continues to push the frontiers of possibility, the fertility landscape is constantly changing, bringing glimmers of hope to those who dare to dream.

As we embark on this journey together, let us approach the challenges of fertility with open hearts and minds.

For inside the pages of this chapter are the keys to unlocking the mysteries that exist within us, guiding us to a greater awareness of ourselves and the wonderful adventure of conception.

So let us jump in, excited and curious, ready to discover the amazing world of reproductive science.

Chapter 2

Lifestyle and Fertility: Making Positive Changes.

In the big tapestry of life, our daily decisions weave the threads that determine our fate. Nowhere is this more clear than in the field of fertility, where our lifestyle can have a significant impact on our ability to create and sustain life.

In this chapter, we go on a voyage of self-discovery, investigating how our daily behaviors and decisions affect our reproductive journey.

Consider a bustling cityscape, where the hustle and bustle of daily life echo through the streets like a symphony of sound.

Here, amidst the clamor of modern living, we find ourselves confronted with choices— choices that can either nourish our bodies and spirits or take us down a part of imbalance and discord.

At the heart of lifestyle and fertility is a delicate mix of nurture and neglect. Our bodies are temples, sophisticated ecosystems designed to thrive in harmony with the environment around us.

However, all too frequently, we find ourselves out of sync, our cycles interrupted by the pressures of modern life.

But don't worry, for inside the confusion comes the possibility of transformation.

By making healthy lifestyle adjustments, we may regain control of our reproductive journey and pave the road for a brighter, more vibrant future.

Let us begin by examining the role of nutrition – the fuel that powers our bodies and nourishes our souls.

In a world saturated with processed foods and artificial additives, it's easy to lose sight of the power of whole, nutrient-dense foods.

Yet, research has shown time and time again that a diet rich in fruits, vegetables, lean proteins, and healthy fats can not only improve fertility but also support overall health and well-being.

But nutrition is just the tip of the iceberg. As we journey deeper into the realm of lifestyle and fertility, we encounter other factors that play a crucial role in shaping our reproductive health.

From the impact of stress and sleep on hormonal balance to the importance of maintaining a healthy weight and exercising regularly, each piece of the puzzle contributes to the larger picture of our fertility journey.

Throughout the chaos and disarray, there remains hope. Every one of us possesses the ability to affect change, rewrite the screenplay of our lives, and begin a journey of transformation.

It may not always be simple, and there will surely be challenges along the path, but with commitment and patience, everything is achievable.

Dear reader, while we travel the meandering paths of lifestyle and fertility, please keep an open heart and mind.

For these pages contain the resources and procedures to help you on your path to conception and beyond.

So, let us embrace the potential for change because the chaos contains the promise of a better tomorrow.

Chapter 3

Nutrition and Fertility: Fueling Your Body for Conception.

In the grand tapestry of life, nutrition serves as the vibrant thread that weaves together the fabric of our existence.

Nowhere is this more evident than in the realm of fertility, where the foods we consume play a pivotal role in shaping our reproductive health and our ability to conceive new life.

In this section, we embark on a journey through the bountiful landscape of nutrition, exploring the power of food to nourish our bodies and fuel our fertility.

Imagine, if you will, a verdant countryside, where fields of golden grain sway gently in the breeze and orchards burst forth with the bounty of the earth.

Here, amidst the abundance of nature's harvest, we find the key to unlocking the secrets of fertility – the nourishing power of whole, nutrient-dense foods.

At the heart of nutrition and fertility lies a simple yet profound truth: the foods we choose to nourish our bodies can have

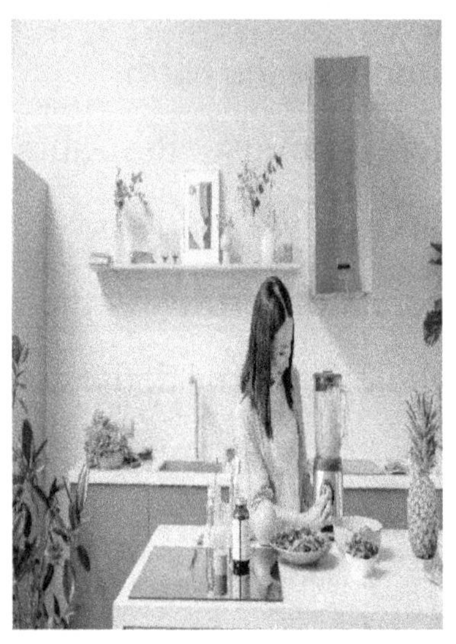

a profound impact on our ability to conceive and carry a child. From the vibrant hues of fresh fruits and vegetables to the rich flavors of whole grains and lean proteins, each bite we take serves to fuel the intricate dance of hormones and processes that govern our reproductive health.

But amidst the abundance of nature's bounty, there lies a landscape fraught with pitfalls and challenges.

In a world inundated with processed foods and artificial additives, it's easy to lose sight of the power of whole, nutrient-dense foods to support fertility.

Yet, research has shown time and time again that a diet rich in fruits, vegetables, whole grains, and lean proteins can not only improve fertility but also support overall health and well-being.

However, nutrition involves more than simply the things we eat; it also includes how we eat them.

In a culture where fast-paced living and convenience frequently take precedence over attentive feeding, it's easy to lose sight of the ancient wisdom of listening to our bodies and respecting their intrinsic knowledge.

However, by slowing down, savoring each meal, and developing a stronger connection with the food we eat, we may harness the healing power of nutrition and assist our fertility journey from the inside out.

As we go more into diet and fertility, we come across additional essential components that have a significant impact on our reproductive health.

From staying hydrated to avoiding dangerous chemicals like alcohol and caffeine to the role of supplements and herbal remedies in supporting fertility, each piece of the puzzle contributes to the larger picture of our fertility journey.

Dear reader, as we explore the beautiful landscape of nutrition and fertility, may we do it with open hearts and minds.

For these pages contain the resources and procedures to help you on your path to conception and beyond.

So, let us embrace the sustaining power of food because its abundance holds the promise of fresh life and a new beginning.

Chapter 4

Stress Management Techniques: Balancing the Mind and Body

Stress reverberates through the air like an unpleasant discord, breaking the harmony of mind, body, and spirit in today's hectic symphony.

Nowhere is this more clear than in the world of fertility, where the constant strains of daily life can cast a pall over our ability to create and nurture life.

In this section, we will go on a voyage of self-discovery, investigating the subtle dance between stress and fertility and discovering the transformational power of stress management practices to restore balance and harmony in our lives.

Imagine, if you will, a peaceful oasis buried within the tumult of the metropolitan environment, where the delicate rustle of leaves and the calming hum of nature We find refuge from the unrelenting pressures of contemporary life here, surrounded by nature's peacefulness, and the opportunity to establish a deeper connection with ourselves and the world around us.

Stress management begins with the realization that stress is not only a mental phenomenon but also a physical and emotional one.

Stress presents itself in a variety of ways, from physical tension to rushing thoughts, each one reflecting the delicate dance between mind and body.

But, despite the chaos, there is a chance for transformation.

By practicing mindfulness and self-awareness, we may begin to unwind from the tangled web of stress that has ensnared us and take control of our internal environment.

Through practices such as meditation, deep breathing, and yoga, we can learn to quiet the restless chatter of the mind and sink into the stillness that lies at the core of our being.

But stress management is more than just finding moments of calm amid commotion; it is also about developing resilience in the face of adversity.

From the ancient wisdom of stoicism to the modern science of positive psychology, there are numerous tools and approaches available to help us develop the mental and emotional fortitude required to weather life's storms with grace and perseverance.

As we delve deeper into stress management, we find other significant aspects that influence our reproductive health.

From the effects of chronic stress on hormone balance to the significance of cultivating good relationships and setting boundaries, each piece of the jigsaw adds to the overall picture of our fertility journey. Dear reader, let us cross the maze of stress and fertility with open hearts and minds. For these pages contain the resources and procedures to help you on your path to conception and beyond. So, let us embrace the transforming potential of stress management because it holds the promise of healing and rebirth.

Chapter 5

Exercise and Fertility: Finding the Right Balance

In the rhythm of life, movement is the throbbing beat that propels us ahead. This is especially evident in the world of fertility, where the ebb and flow of physical activity may mold our bodies and brains, as well as influence our ability to conceive and raise children.

In this chapter, we'll take a journey through the rich landscape of exercise, investigating the transforming power of movement to promote fertility and overall well-being.

Imagine a beautiful forest glade, where dappled sunshine penetrates through the canopy above, casting dancing shadows on the forest floor.

Here, among the melody of birdsong and the rustle of leaves, we discover ourselves called to movement – to dance, to stretch, to run wild and free.

At the heart of exercise and fertility is a delicate balance of action and rest, of pushing our bodies to new heights while also respecting their need for repair and regeneration.

From the rhythmic cadence of a brisk stroll to the exhilarating rush of a heart-pounding workout, every movement we make helps to nourish our bodies and souls while also supporting our reproductive journey.

However, in the middle of a cacophony of contradictory advice and perspectives, it is easy to lose sight of the fundamental essence of exercise moving with joy and intention, and honoring our bodies' particular requirements.

Whether you find consolation in the calm flow of yoga, the uplifting beauty of dance, or the thrilling rush of outdoor adventure, the key is to find what brings you joy and fulfillment and embrace it with open arms.

But exercise is more than simply physical activity; it's also about developing a stronger connection with ourselves and the world around us.

Through techniques like mindfulness and body awareness, we can learn to listen to our bodies' subtle hints and acknowledge their intrinsic wisdom as we move through the world.

As we delve deeper into the topic of exercise and fertility, we come across other significant aspects that influence our reproductive health.

From the effect of hard exercise on hormonal balance to the importance of striking a

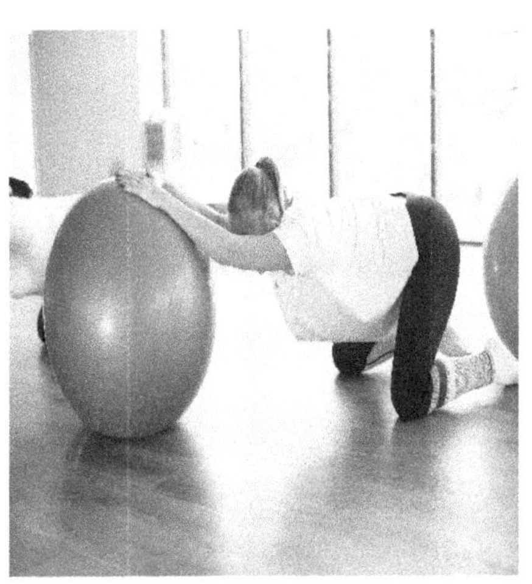

balance in our fitness routines and avoiding extremes, each piece of the puzzle adds to the overall picture of our reproductive journey.

Dear reader, as we explore the vivid landscape of fitness and conception, may we do so with open hearts and minds.

For these pages contain the resources and procedures to help you on your path to conception and beyond.

So, embrace the transforming power of movement, since it holds the promise of life, joy, and increased fertility.

Chapter 6

Fertility Myths Debunked: Separating Fact from Fiction

Myths and falsehoods swirl across the enormous tapestry of human knowledge, clouding our comprehension of the world around us.

This is particularly evident in the area of reproduction, where centuries-old ideas and obsolete notions continue to affect our views and impact our decisions.

In this section, we'll go on a myth-busting adventure, separating reality from fiction and discovering the truth about common reproductive misconceptions.

Imagine a beautiful night with shadows dancing on the walls and whispers of ancient wisdom filling the air.

Here, in the solitude of the night, we find ourselves confronted with the ghosts of fertility myths past—tales of superstition and misperception that have lingered in the collective consciousness for generations.

Fertility myths include a kernel of truth that has been perverted and expanded throughout time to bear little similarity to reality.

These beliefs, which range from the idea that certain sexual positions can influence conception to the belief that women are most fertile during ovulation, persist despite evidence to the contrary.

But don't worry, since inside the shadows lurks the light of knowledge, ready to illuminate the gloom and remove the myths that obscure our understanding of fertility. Let us begin by looking at one of the most common myths: that aging only influences a woman's fertility.

While age has a substantial impact on fertility in both men and women, it is not the only determining factor. fertility is impacted

by a myriad of factors, including genetics, lifestyle, and overall health.

Another frequent fallacy that persists is that infertility is only a female issue.

In actuality, infertility affects men and women equally, with male factor infertility accounting for roughly one-third of all instances.

However, the stigma around male infertility lingers, causing many to suffer in silence and delaying treatment.

Perhaps the most devastating fallacy of all is that infertility is a personal failing, a reflection of one's human worth. Infertility, like any other medical issue, requires compassion, understanding, and support.

By breaking down the barriers of shame and stigma, we can create a culture of empathy and inclusivity, empowering individuals to seek the help they need without fear or judgment.

As we go deeper into fertility myths, we come across other beliefs that impact our thoughts and influence our decisions. From the misconception that stress causes infertility to the notion that certain foods or rituals might improve fertility, each myth emphasizes the importance of critical thinking and evidence-based decision-making.

As we travel the maze of fertility myths, please keep an open heart and mind. For these pages contain the resources and procedures to help you on your path to conception and beyond. So, let us embrace the truth and eliminate the myths that veil our understanding of fertility, because the light of knowledge holds the promise of clarity, understanding, and empowerment in decision-making.

Chapter 7

Fertility Tracking Methods: Tools to Understand Your Cycle

The delicate dance of the menstrual cycle holds the key to understanding the ebb and flow of fertility.

Nowhere is this more clear than in fertility tracking, where contemporary technology and traditional wisdom combine to empower people on their path to conception.

In this chapter, we'll take a tour through the moon's cycles and the body's rhythms, looking at the numerous fertility tracking tools available and discovering the insights they bring into our reproductive health.

Imagine a peaceful lakeside at dawn, with the water shimmering like liquid gold beneath the rising sun. In the silence of the morning, we are drawn to the gentle regularity of the waves, which represent the cycles that regulate our bodies and lives.

At the heart of fertility tracking is a simple yet profound truth: knowledge is power. Understanding the various indications and patterns of our menstrual cycle allows us to unlock fertility secrets and get insight into our 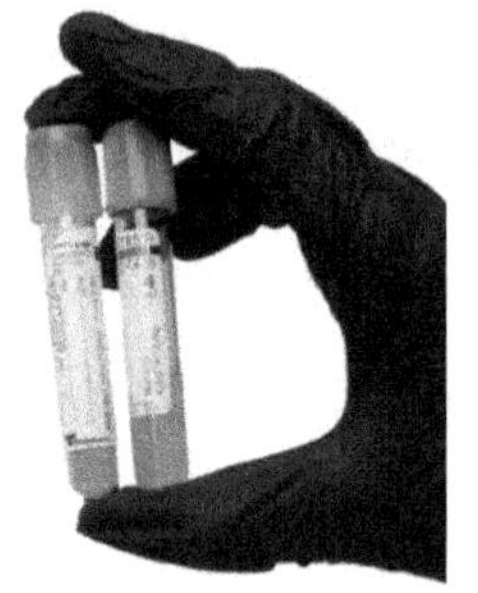 bodies' complicated workings. From the rise and fall of basal body temperature to changes in cervical mucous and cervix position, each signal is a piece of the puzzle that guides us on our journey to conception.

However, fertility tracking is more than just collecting statistics; it's also about building a closer connection to ourselves and our bodies. Charting, writing, and meditation are all techniques that can help us learn to listen to our bodies' subtle messages and acknowledge their intrinsic wisdom as we navigate the world.

As we delve deeper into the world of fertility tracking, we come across a plethora of tools and procedures, each with its unique insights about our reproductive health.

From the traditional wisdom of the fertility awareness method to the modern convenience of ovulation predictor kits and fertility monitoring apps, there are numerous resources available to assist us on our journey.

Despite the multitude of alternatives, it's crucial to realize that fertility tracking isn't a one-size-fits-all method. What works for one person may not work for another, so it's critical to choose the strategy that most truly resonates with your specific requirements and preferences.

Dear reader, while we negotiate the meandering paths of fertility tracking, let us keep an open heart and mind.

For these pages contain the resources and procedures to help you on your path to conception and beyond. So, let us embrace our body's rhythms and the moon's cycles, for they hold the potential for comprehension, insight, and empowered decision-making.

Chapter 8

Natural Remedies and Supplements For Enhancing Fertility

Naturally Nature's Garden of Life provides a plethora of healing solutions that patiently await discovery and welcome.

Nowhere is this more clear than in the field of fertility, where traditional wisdom and modern science combine to provide a treasure mine of natural therapies and supplements to promote reproductive health. In this chapter, we'll take a journey across the rich terrain of botanicals and nutrients, investigating nature's ability to boost fertility and foster new life.

Imagine a sun-kissed meadow where wildflowers grow in a riot of color and the air is thick with the aroma of earth and sky.

We find ourselves here, surrounded by the splendor of nature's riches drawn to the healing power of plants – a source of nourishment and vitality for body, mind, and soul.

At the heart of natural treatments and supplements is a deep respect for the earth's wisdom and the

human body's innate healing ability.

From the soft embrace of herbal teas to the strong extracts of adaptogenic herbs, each

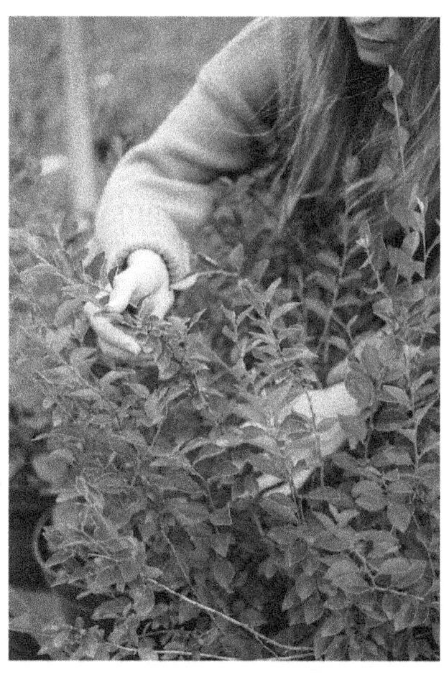

therapy provides its distinct combination of nutrients and chemicals to promote reproductive health and conception.

However, natural treatments and supplements do more than just relieve symptoms; they also address the underlying causes of imbalances and promote the

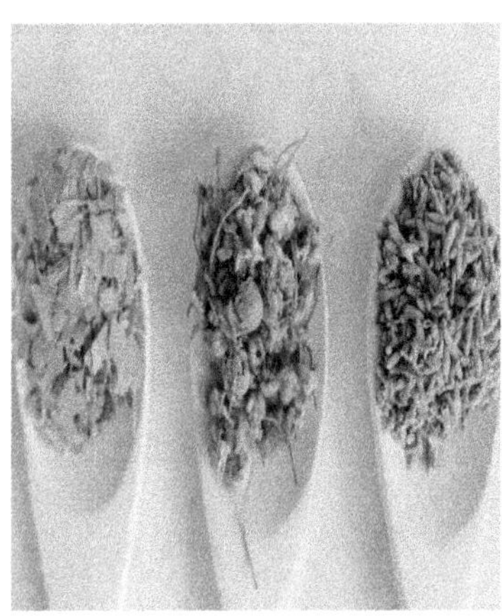

body's natural ability to repair itself. Whether you're dealing with hormone imbalances, inflammation, or oxidative stress, there are a variety of botanicals and nutrients that can help restore balance and harmony to your reproductive system.

As we delve deeper into the world of natural cures and supplements, we face a plethora of possibilities, each with its own set of advantages and potential adverse effects.

From vitex and maca root to coenzyme Q10 and omega-3 fatty acids, the possibilities are limitless - but it's critical to approach supplements

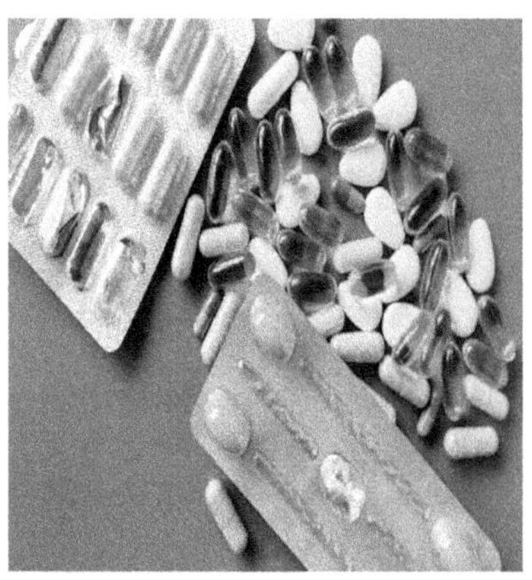

with caution and mindfulness, and to check with a healthcare expert before adding any new treatments to your routine.

However, amid so many alternatives, it's crucial to remember that natural therapies and supplements are only one part of the reproductive jigsaw.

Lifestyle factors including nutrition, stress management, and exercise play a critical influence in determining reproductive health,

therefore it's important to address these parts of your life in conjunction 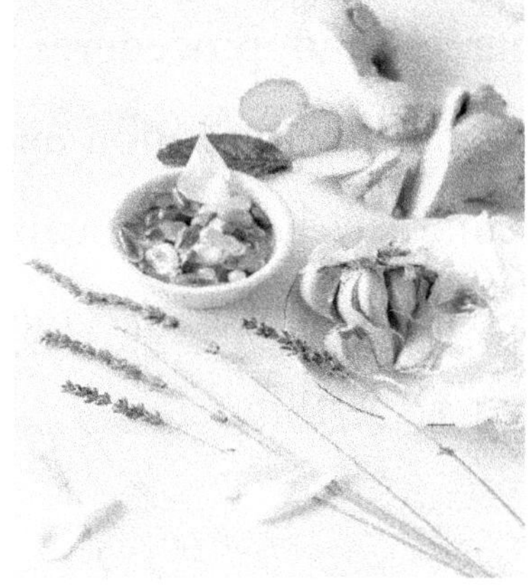 with any natural remedies or supplements you may be considering.

Dear reader, as we explore the verdant terrain of natural treatments and supplements, may we do so with open hearts and minds. For these pages contain the resources and procedures to help you on your path to conception and beyond. So, let us embrace nature's healing force, which holds the promise of vigor, harmony, and increased fertility.

Chapter 9

Seeking Professional Help: When to Consult a Fertility Specialist

In the delicate fabric of fertility, there are times when the route ahead appears unknown,

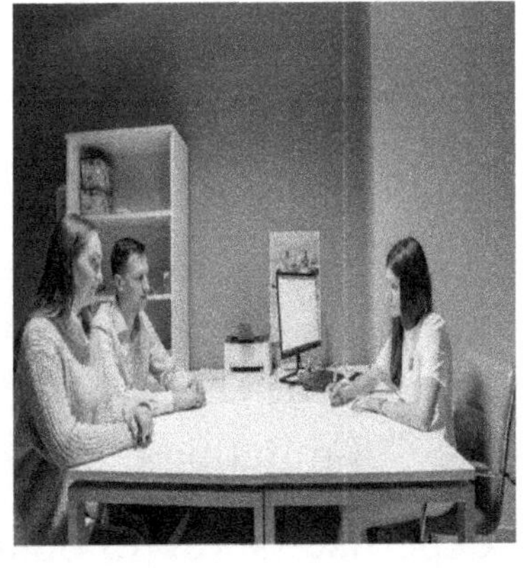

veiled in shadows of doubt and anxiety. During these moments, the advice and skills of a fertility specialist can serve as a beacon of hope, illuminating the path to understanding, healing, and, eventually, realizing one's goals of parenting.

In this chapter, we'll take a look at the signals that it's time to seek the advice of a fertility specialist, as well as the measures to take once you've decided to speak with one.

Imagine a bustling cityscape, accentuated by the spires of towering buildings, each one a symbol of human intellect and aspiration. Amidst the rush and bustle of urban life, we are presented with the complexities of fertility - a landscape plagued with problems and hurdles, but also filled with moments of success and hope.

Recognizing the limitations of our knowledge and expertise is key to obtaining professional aid. While we may do a lot to help our fertility journey with lifestyle modifications, natural remedies, and self-care practices, there are times when the advice of a skilled specialist is required to navigate the complexity of reproductive health. But how do you know when it's time to see a fertility specialist? Numerous indicators suggest the need for professional help, ranging from trouble conceiving despite regular, unprotected intercourse to recurrent pregnancy loss, irregular menstrual cycles, or underlying health issues that may affect fertility. If you are experiencing any of these issues, it may be time to consult a reproductive professional.

Once you've decided to see a fertility expert, the next step is to discover the proper one for you. This could include investigating different clinics and practitioners in your region, reading reviews, and seeking referrals from friends, family, or your primary care physician. It's crucial to select a service that not only has the knowledge and experience to meet your specific requirements but he or she is also someone you can trust and rely on.

As you begin your journey with a fertility specialist, keep an open mind and a desire to collaborate.

Your fertility specialist will collaborate with you to undertake a comprehensive evaluation of your reproductive health, which may involve a review of your medical

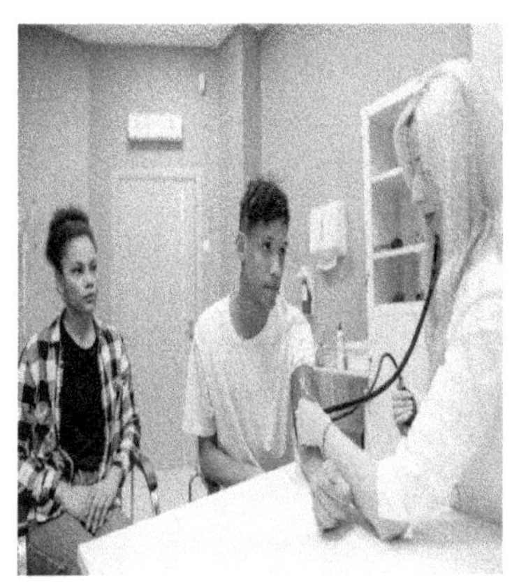

history, physical exams, and diagnostic procedures like blood work, imaging investigations, or fertility testing.

After a diagnosis is made, your fertility specialist will collaborate with you to create a personalized treatment plan based on your specific requirements and circumstances.

This could include lifestyle changes, medication, surgical treatments, and assisted reproductive technologies as depending on the root cause of your fertility issues, you may need intrauterine insemination (IUI), in vitro fertilization (IVF), or other therapies. However, getting professional assistance is more than just solving a problem; it is also about obtaining support and direction along the road. Your fertility specialist will accompany you on your journey, providing support, empathy, and expertise along the way.

Dear reader, while you negotiate the labyrinth of fertility, remember you are not alone. Within the realm of fertility specialists, there is a wealth of information, competence, and compassion waiting to guide you on your path to conception and beyond.

So, let us accept the wisdom and advice of these dedicated professionals because under their care lies the promise of understanding, healing, and the realization of your dreams of parenthood.

Chapter 10

Emotional Support Throughout the Fertility Journey

In the complicated dance of fertility, emotions flow like currents through a huge ocean,

altering 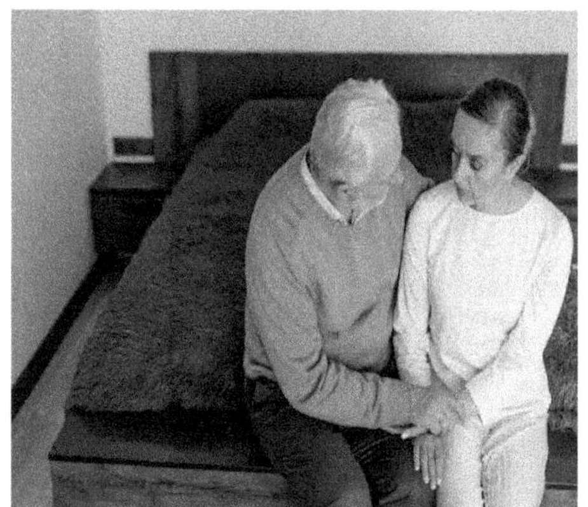 our

experiences and coloring our impressions of the world around us.

This is particularly noticeable during the reproductive journey, where the highs of optimism and anticipation are quickly followed by the lows of disappointment and despair.

In this chapter, we'll take a journey through the emotional landscape, learning about the value of emotional support and resilience during the reproductive journey, as well as ways for navigating the highs and lows with grace.

Imagine a moonlit night, where the stars glitter like diamonds against the velvet sky, and the air is thick with the aroma of jasmine and lavender.

Here, in the solitude of the night, we are confronted with the rawness of our emotions - a kaleidoscope of joy, anguish, fear, and longing that ebbs and flows with the tide.

At the heart of the fertility journey is an awareness of the enormous impact that emotions may have on our physical and mental health. From the exhilarating surge of joy at the start of a new cycle to the crushing weight of sorrow when a pregnancy test comes back negative, each feeling serves as a mirror, reflecting the depths of our longing and the heights of our expectations.

However, in the middle of emotional turmoil, there is an opportunity for growth and transformation.

By developing self-awareness and compassion, We may learn to handle the ups and downs of the fertility journey with grace and fortitude. We may create a space for reflection and healing by engaging in practices like mindfulness, meditation, and journaling, allowing ourselves to recognize the entire range of emotions that come along the path.

However, emotional support is more than simply self-care; it also includes reaching out to others for support and connection. Whether it's a trustworthy friend, a supportive partner, or a professional counselor, having someone to lean on during stressful times can make all the difference. By sharing our problems and victories with others, we may foster a sense of belonging and community that will see us through even the darkest days.

As we delve deeper into the world of emotional support, we come across more critical components that play an important part in molding our resilience and well-being.

Each piece of the puzzle, from the need to set boundaries and practice self-compassion to the healing power of creativity and expression, adds to the overall picture of emotional health and resilience.

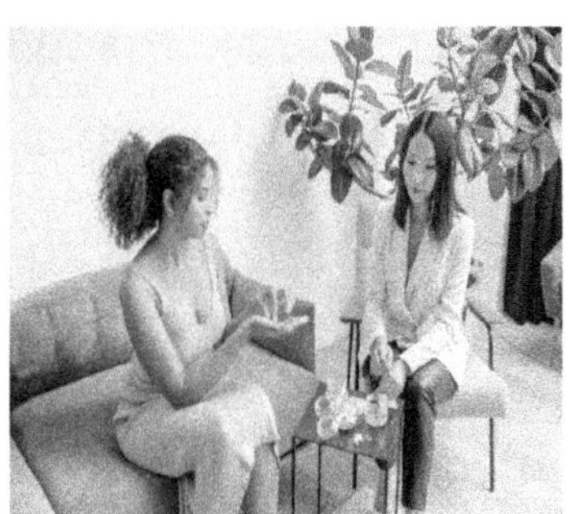

Dear reader, while you sail the turbulent seas of the fertility journey, remember that you are not alone. Within the depths of your own heart, you will find the wisdom and strength to weather any storm, and the embrace of others will provide you with support and connection to keep you going. So, let us accept the richness of our emotions, because inside its depths is the promise of healing growth and resilience.

Chapter 11

Case Studies: True Stories of Overcoming Fertility Obstacles

In the broad fabric of human experience, each of us carries a tale within us - a narrative of triumphs and sufferings, hopes and dreams, difficulties and successes. Nowhere is this more clear than in the area of fertility, where the path to pregnancy is as distinct and individual as the people who begin.

In this section, we will delve into the personal tales of real-life people who have suffered fertility issues and discover the lessons, insights, and inspiration they may provide.

Imagine, if you will, a quiet cafe tucked in the center of a busy city, where the air is filled with the rich perfume of freshly made coffee and A pleasant murmur of discourse. We are drawn to the stories that remain in the spaces between us, stories of hope and resilience, love and loss, perseverance and triumph, amidst the warmth and camaraderie of both friends and strangers.

At the center of each case study is a real individual, complete with hopes and dreams, fears and doubts, pleasures and tragedies. Through their stories, we gain insight into the breadth of their experiences and the richness of their parenting path.

Consider the case of Sarah and James, a couple who struggled with infertility for years before becoming pregnant through in vitro fertilization (IVF). Their journey was plagued by innumerable setbacks and disappointments, including failed reproductive treatments to the headache of miscarriage. Despite this, they stayed persistent in their quest to become parents, and their dedication was rewarded

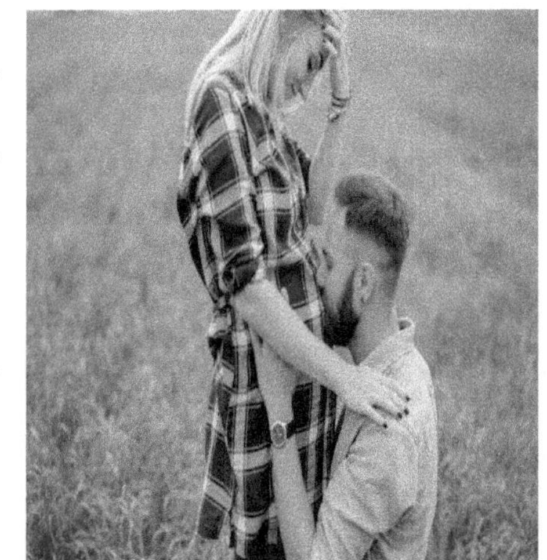

when they welcomed their long-awaited miracle into the world.

Consider the example of Michael, a single man who chose surrogacy after being diagnosed with male factor infertility. His journey was plagued with difficulties and doubts, from navigating the intricate legal and ethical issues surrounding surrogacy to dealing with his own emotions of inadequacy and self-doubt.

Throughout it all, he found strength and resilience in the love and support of his family and friends, as well as the knowledge that he was making progress toward his ambition of being a parent.

However, not all fertility journeys end happily, and for every success tale, countless others involve grief and loss.

Consider the story of Emily and David, a couple who encountered the heartbreaking reality of recurrent pregnancy loss on their journey to fatherhood.

Despite their best efforts and the constant support of their medical team, they were unable to bring a baby to term and had to make the tough decision to seek adoption instead.

As we progress through the case studies, we come across a wide range of situations, each of which demonstrates the tenacity of the human spirit and the ability of love and hope to overcome even the most difficult circumstances. From the triumph of successful fertility treatments to the pain of miscarriage and pregnancy loss, each story serves as a reminder of the fertility journey's complexity and unpredictability, as well as the value of compassion, empathy, and support along the road.

Dear reader, as you immerse yourself in the experiences of these brave individuals, may you find comfort in knowing that you are not alone on your path to parenting.

For inside the pages of these case studies is the wisdom, inspiration, and hope that will guide you through even the darkest of days and illuminate the path to the realization of your goals. So, let us respect the richness of these stories, as well as the human spirit's resiliency, which shines brightly inside them.

Chapter 12

Moving Forward: Empowering Yourself Beyond the Fertility Journey.

Every ending in life's maze is also a beginning, a portal to new possibilities, adventures, and horizons waiting to be discovered.

This is especially evident in the reproductive journey, where the desire for parenthood is only one chapter in our lives' wider tale.

In this final chapter, we will go on a journey of reflection and empowerment, exploring how we can move forward with courage, resilience, and optimism, regardless of the outcome of our fertility journey.

Imagine, if you will, a mountainside at sunrise, where the air is clean and clear, and the world stretches out before you in all its glory and splendor. Amidst the beauty and majesty of the natural world, we are filled with awe and wonder - a reminder of the endless possibilities that exist within each of us, ready to be explored and embraced.

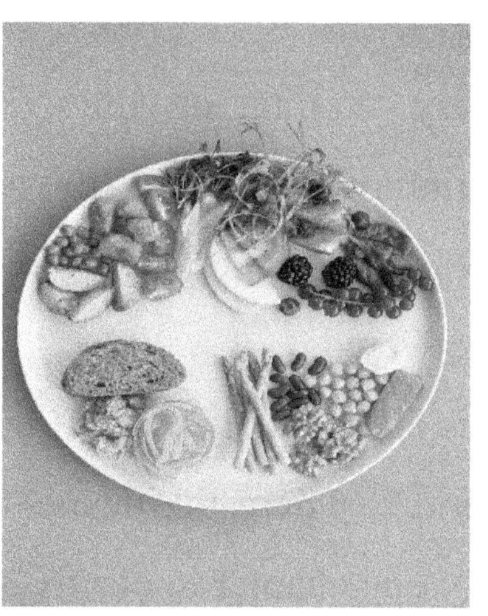

Moving forward requires recognizing the power of resilience - the ability to adapt and grow in the face of adversity, emerging from even the darkest of days with newfound strength and purpose.

While the reproductive journey may be filled with failures and hardships, it is also an opportunity for growth and transformation, as well as a reminder of the human spirit's tenacity.

However, going ahead is more than just resilience; it is also about empowerment. It is about taking ownership of our lives and our choices and embracing the freedom to create the future we desire, regardless of the obstacles we may face along the way. Whether it's pursuing alternate paths to parenting like adoption or surrogacy, or finding joy and meaning in other areas of our lives, several opportunities are waiting to be explored outside of the reproductive journey.

As we delve deeper into the domain of progress, we come across other fundamental ideas that might lead us on our path. From self-care and self-compassion to gratitude and mindfulness, every step we take toward empowerment takes us closer to living a life of purpose and fulfillment, regardless of the outcome of our reproductive journey.

But arguably the most crucial element of all is the power of connection - the understanding that we are not alone on this path and that we are stronger when we band together in the community and support one another.

Whether it's reaching out to friends and family for support, seeking the advice of a therapist or support group, or connecting with others who have been through a similar experience, there is strength in solidarity and comfort in knowing we are not alone.

Dear reader, as you approach a fresh beginning, may you embrace the adventure ahead with courage, resilience, and hope. For in the depths of your own heart resides the wisdom and strength to manage even the most difficult of paths, and within the embrace of others lies the support and connection to sustain you along the way. So, let us step forward together, with open hearts and open minds, and embrace the infinite possibilities that lie within each of us.

Conclusion

As we near the end of our transforming journey through the complexities of fertility, we are reminded that every step we take, and every decision we make, demonstrates the resilience of the human spirit and the power of hope to guide us through even the darkest of days. In the pages of this book, we've delved into the secrets of conception and the complexity of the reproductive journey, as well as the depths of our longing and dreams. Along the journey, we have faced moments of triumph and failure, periods of joy and sorrow—each one a

thread woven into the rich tapestry of our
life.

But, despite the twists and turns of the

fertility problem, there is one common thread that connects us all: the thread of hope. Hope is what keeps us going in our darkest hours,

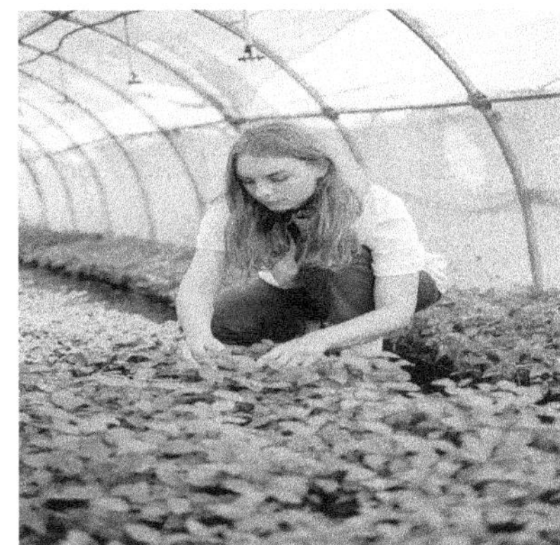

whispering words of encouragement and inspiration when everything seems lost. Hope nourishes our resilience, providing us with the courage to pick ourselves up and persevere in the face of hardship. And it is hope that propels us forward on our journey, illuminating the route ahead and highlighting the possibilities that are within reach.

As we reflect on the lessons learned and insights obtained along the road, we are reminded that the fertility struggle is not only about the goal, but also about the voyage itself is a path of self-discovery, empowerment, and compassion.

It is a voyage that invites us to embrace the full breadth of our experiences, both the highs and the lows, and to seek meaning and purpose in the face of ambiguity and doubt.

But, perhaps most importantly, the fertility challenge is a voyage of connection, reminding us of the power of community and the significance of reaching out to others for help and understanding.

Whether it's a friend's consoling embrace, the advice of a trusted healthcare expert, or the unity of a support group, we are reminded that we are not alone on this road and that we may find strength and solace in each other's company.

As we say goodbye to the pages of this book and move forth into the unknown, may we carry with us the lessons learned and wisdom gained, knowing that we are stronger and more resilient for having ventured on this adventure. Let us face the challenges ahead with courage and commitment, knowing that we can mold our destiny and create the future we want.

And let us never underestimate the power of hope, the guiding light that shines within each of us, illuminating the way to healing, satisfaction, and joy. For inside the depths of our hearts is the boundless potential to dream, hope, and trust in the possibility of miracles—and it is this belief that will propel us ahead on our road to a future full of love, laughter, and fresh starts.

So, dear reader, as you flip the final page of this book and begin the next chapter of your life, may you do so with an open heart and mind, ready to face both the challenges and the joys that await you. And may you never forget the journey that led you to this point - the reproductive struggle, and the important lessons it has to teach us all.

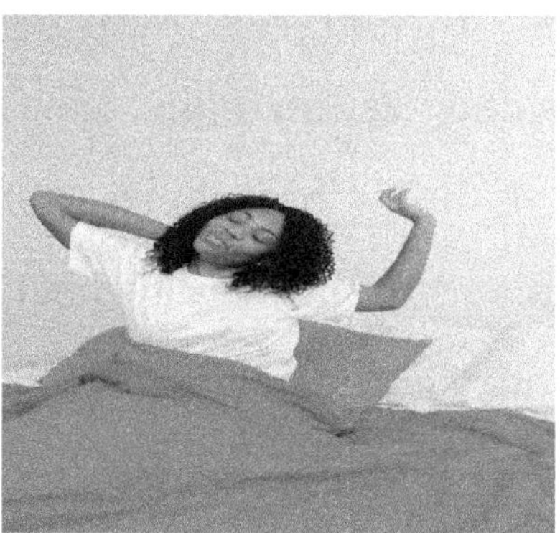

www.ingramcontent.com/pod-product-compliance
Lightning Source LLC
Chambersburg PA
CBHW072338270726
48659CB00022B/1893